OIL
&
WATER

HOW TO CARE
FOR AFRICAN-AMERICAN HAIR

BY KIA SPRINKLE

1st Edition 2023

Dedication

This book is dedicated to all of my beautiful nieces:

Marshay, Alley, Trenekia, Ashley, Amena, Lexi, Sian, Naava, Amorie, Maxi, MacKenzie, and Ella.

And, to all the black women and girls who struggle with taking care of their hair. Not only do we struggle with doing our hair but we struggle with accepting our hair. We are constantly told and shown in society that beautiful hair is long, flowing, and straight. Quite the opposite of ours. We don't have flowing, straight hair and so many black women oftentimes feel unbeautiful because of this. We feel the need to conform with society and also within our community. All women desire to be beautiful. The most beautiful women get the best men, the best husband, the best house, the best friends, the best life. And so, we too, black women, are in the race for supreme beauty thus having supreme success in life. It is difficult being born into societies that do not deem your look as the standard of beauty. However, we must stop conforming and start transforming back into the beauty standard that God created for US. We are beautiful. Our hair is beautiful. And we can redefine the beauty standard if we simply do not conform.

Table of Contents

1
Lines & Circles

*L*ines and Circles. Lines and Circles. What am I talking about? I am describing the shapes of hair. Lines and Circles. Straight lines, wavy lines, and varied circles. Hair grows from our heads and all over our bodies in either a line or a circle. For most people of European descent, their hairs grow in a line. And for most people of African descent, their hairs grow in a circle. Most African-Americans are mixed with African and European ancestry and therefore have hair that grows in a circle. The width and tightness or looseness of our circles vary from person to person and depend on the percentage of line and circle hair combination in our bloodline.

Circles, like lines, are a very common occurrence in nature. Circles or spheres are abundant in nature and our universe. They are seen in planets, stars, celestial bodies, tree rings, raindrops, oceans, to name a few. Thus, we know that the circles growing from our heads have been naturally created too. I want all African-Americans to know that our circle hair is a natural occurrence in nature. God created our hair. This fact is important due to the misrepresentation of circle hair in marketing and media. Due to the adverse and violent history of America, people with circle hair and dark skin have legally and socially been oppressed for financial exploitation and advancement of the country. Because of this, a negative connotation of circle hair has surely seeped into the consciousness of most Americans, including those of us with circle hair. These negative inner feelings make us think and act a certain way about our hair and this is why you see a large percentage of African-Americans walking around with lined hair wigs on. Most times, this isn't comfortable but because of the beauty standards and the need to be socially acceptable, women, especially women of African descent choose to be seen with line hair. This subtle acceptance doesn't apply to African Americans alone, but also to many other colonized countries as well. However, for this book, I will be specifically speaking on what I know as an American. I want to stress to African Americans that the circle hair growing from our heads, IS A NATURAL OCCURANCE IN NATURE. Line hair is also a natural occurrence in nature but not on the heads of people of African descent. Once we fully accept seeing ourselves with our circle hair in its natural state, the whole world will have no choice but to accept it too.

These points are important before I begin my discussion on our hair care because the more you can accept your hair as a natural and beautiful part of nature the easier it will be for you to want to work to take care of it. Yes, our hair takes work, just like all other hair. Yes, it is harder to take care of circle hair than line hair. Yes, I know it seems harsh. Life is hard and our hair is difficult too?! I promise good does come to those who work hard toward a particular goal in life.

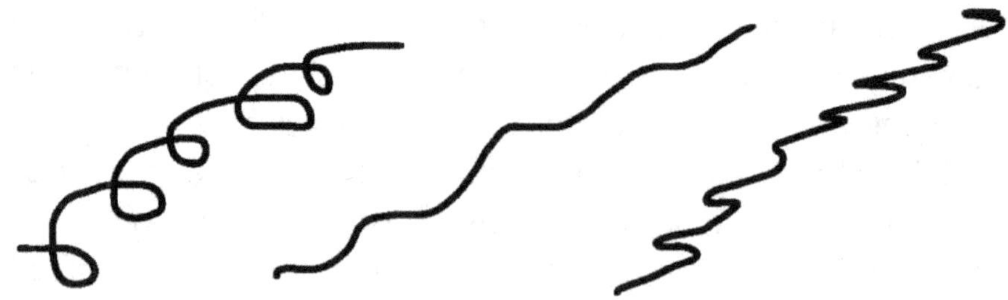

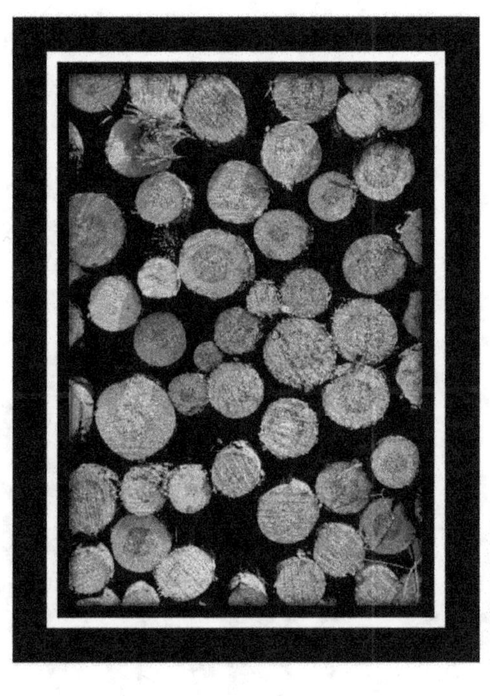

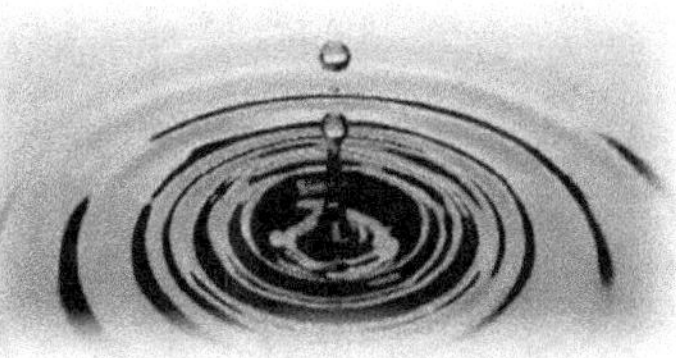

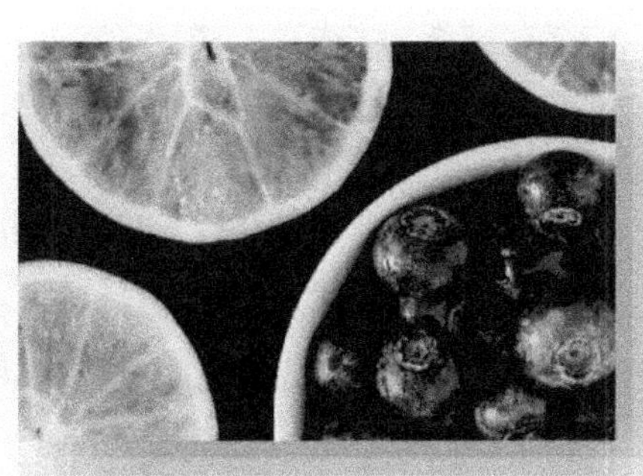

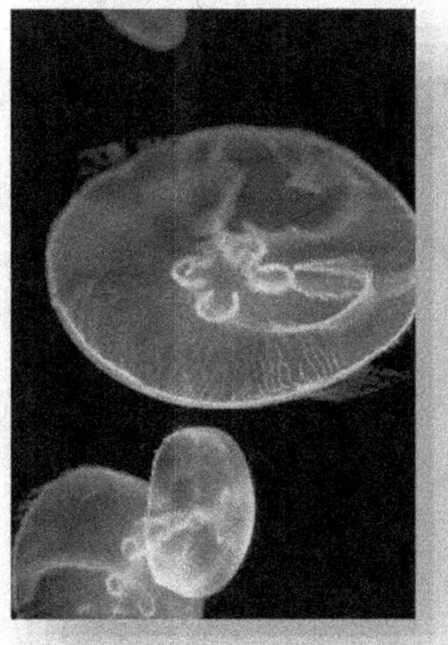

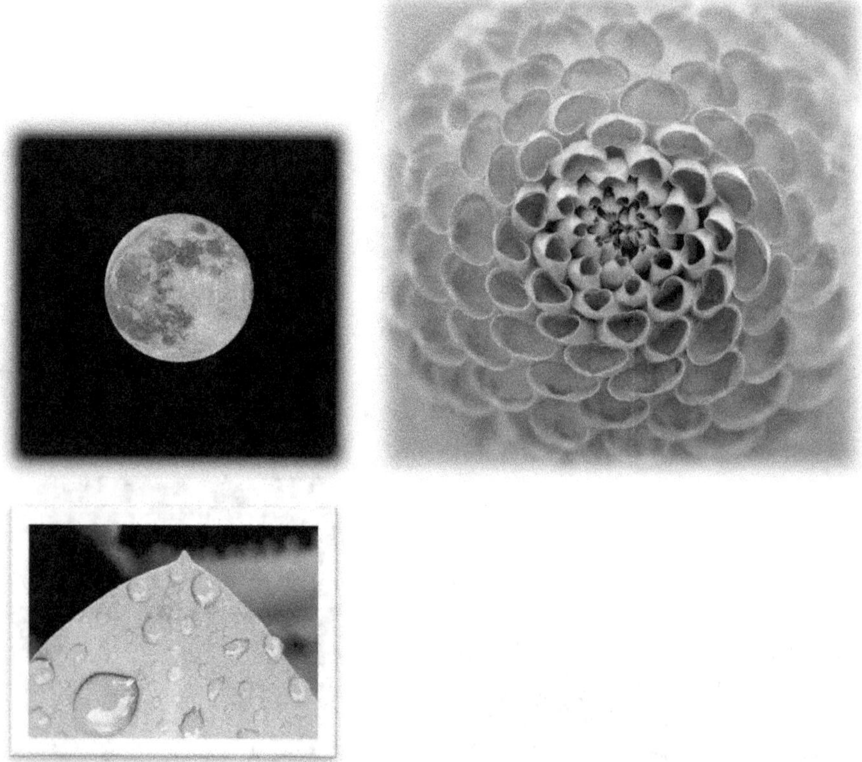

2
The Method That Works

*Y*ou must love your body before deciding to eat in a way that will keep it healthy. You have to accept and love yourself before you can communicate boundaries and standards that would be conducive to a healthy and loving relationship. And, you must love your circle hair and accept it for what it is before you will do what is necessary to take care of it.

I have written this book to try to convince you all to take care of your circle hair. Your hair is important! Why? You ask. Simply because it **feels** good to have healthy circle hair. Because without healthy, maintained hair we are limiting our expression as an individual and culturally.

There are many YouTubers and books out there that can explain the science of what I am about to tell you. This book will explain my knowledge from 10-plus years of experience with my own hair through trial and error and **feeling** what is right. Feeling. There's that word again. African- Americans and all people of African descent have extraordinarily strong and intuitive feelings and emotions. Methods and systems are important and necessary. Likewise, methods and systems are perfected through feelings. I will explain the method that works best for our hair. However, I am explaining the method to use so that you can "feel" good about your hair and yourself. Because our feelings are our gift as a culture. Our feelings have taken us far as African-Americans. The strength we conjure through our feelings and emotions and our ability to create and adapt through them is the reason we are still here in America and still a strong people today and will be forever. OUR FEELINGS MATTER. This method of caring for our hair is meant to help us **feel good** about ourselves. Truly and deeply. Our feelings create our experiences which in turn create our reality. Our collective feelings are powerful and transformative. Our collective good feelings about ourselves and our love for ourselves will create the energy to be recompensed on Earth. I will start with our hair.

There is a basic method to taking care of the average African-American head of hair. The two best ingredients of the method are oil and water. When it comes to our hair, oil and water do mix. That's what creates the magic!

3
The Basics

*O*ur hair needs oils and water to thrive, grow and be healthy.

Oil- Any of numerous unctuous combustible substances that are liquid or can be liquefied easily on warming, are soluble in ether but not in water, and leave a greasy stain on paper or cloth. Merriam-Webster definition.

Water- The liquid that descends from the clouds as rain, forms streams, lakes, and seas, and is a major constituent of all living matter and that when pure is an odorless, tasteless, very slightly compressible liquid oxide of hydrogen H_2O which appears bluish in thick layers, freezes at 0° C and boils at 100° C, has a maximum density at 4° C and high specific heat, is feebly ionized to hydrogen and hydroxyl ions, and is a poor conductor of electricity and a good solvent. Merriam- Webster definition.

There are many different oils that you can use in your hair and although there is no substitute for water there are different water-based creams that will work on our hair as well.

Examples of good oils: Olive oil, avocado oil, grapeseed oil, sunflower oil, jojoba oil, petroleum

Examples of good water: Water, tap water, bottled water, distilled water, and water-based creams (the first ingredient is water).

Hair Porosity

Essentially, hair porosity is <u>**your hair's ability to absorb and**</u>

retain moisture. The porosity of your hair affects how well oils and moisture pass throughout the outermost layer of your hair, known as the cuticle.

Low porosity hair has cuticles that are bound very close together, normal porosity hair has cuticles that are slightly less bound, and high porosity hair has cuticles that are more widely spread out.

Low porosity hair is characterized by a tightly bound cuticle layer, making it difficult for moisture to penetrate, and also difficult for moisture to escape once it has penetrated the hair. Low porosity hair is characterized by hair that takes a long time to dry, can be resistant to colouring and other chemical processes, and is prone to product build-up.

On the other hand, **high porosity hair** has gaps and openings in the cuticle layer, allowing moisture to easily pass in and out. Highly porous hair typically dries quickly, is prone to frizz, and can tend towards feeling dry.

There are a few quick tests that are popular for people to conduct at home to determine the porosity level of their hair. These tests are not guaranteed to give an exact result however they will certainly help you understand how porosity works.

The Float Test:
- Take some strands of hair from your brush or comb (be sure to use clean hair as products can alter the results) and drop them into a glass of water
- Let them sit for a few minutes, and if the strands float after the time is up, you likely have low-porosity hair. If it sinks, the hair is likely to be high porosity
- If the hair floats somewhere in the middle of the glass, this would indicate medium porosity hair.

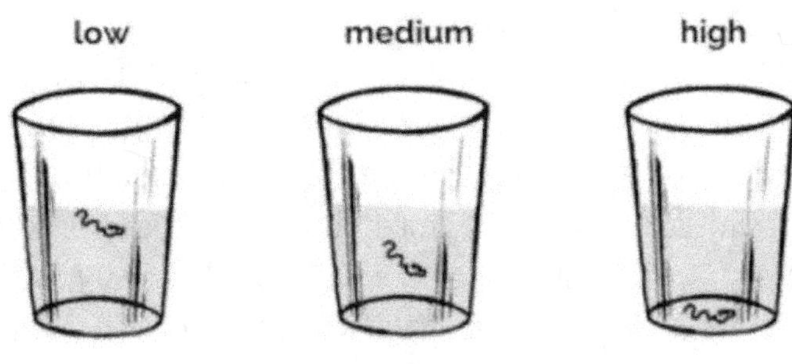

the FLOAT test

Image source: naturallclub.com

The Spray Bottle Test:
- Take a small section of your hair and mist it with some water from a spray bottle.
- Watch closely, if the water beads up on the hair, it is **low porosity**
- If the water absorbs quickly, the hair is **high porosity**
- If you notice the water sitting on the hair for a couple of minutes before absorbing in, the hair is **medium porosity**

Why is Porosity Important?
It is important to know your hair porosity to help you identify what products work best on your hair. Oil and water are all we need on our hair but the specific oils and moisture products that work best for your hair are particular to your curl pattern and porosity. Knowing your hair type helps you to take the best care of your hair.

Styling
LOC and LCO Methods
Two methods work best for keeping our circle/curly hair moisturized, LOC and LCO. LOC stands for Liquid first, Oil second, and Cream last. LCO stands for Liquid first, Cream second, and Oil last. The method that works best for your hair will most likely have to do with the porosity of your hair. But you will have to experiment to know for sure.

Should I use the LOC Method?
Those with high porosity hair should use the LOC Method. Retaining moisture is super important since high porosity has a very open cuticle, meaning it can easily lose moisture. You want to start with liquid (water or a spray leave-in) just to hydrate your tresses. Next, you want to add oil to seal. Lastly, you should apply a cream or butter onto the hair strands. The reason why cream should be the last step for high porosity hair is because it has the thickest consistency, meaning it'll hold in moisture.

Should I use the LCO Method?
For our low porosity naturals, I recommend the LCO Method. Follow the sequence of liquid, cream, and oil. Low porosity has a tight, almost shut cuticle and that's why it's important to add liquid first, cream second to moisturize, and oil last to seal in moisture. Doing it in this sequence will allow moisture to penetrate deeply into the hair shaft, which is critical for low-porosity hair since it tends to repel moisture.

If you have normal porosity, you can choose whatever method you want. Both should work perfectly fine on your hair since your cuticle isn't too tight or too loose.

Basic Hair Tools
Some hair tools work best with curly hair. Here are the tools you will need to make your styling easier.

- Wide Tooth Comb (rounded teeth)
- Good quality medium tooth comb
- Fingers to comb through hair (file those nails)
- Small spray bottle for water
- Plastic cap for deep conditioning
- Silk (not satin) bonnet or pillow case to sleep on
- Patience and Time

4
My Hair Story

*H*ello, my name is Kia and I have low porosity curly type 4 hair. I'm a circle hair girl and I am African- American. I first cut all my permed hair off when I was about twenty-six years old. I was living in Washington, DC at the time and it felt like everyone was natural in DC. So, after I made that decision, I didn't feel very awkward or out of place in public. However, the day I cut all of my hair off to about two inches I looked in the mirror and felt weird and ugly, for a moment. It was a shock! It didn't look like the person staring at me from the mirror was me. Without wasting much time, I quickly went to a braid shop and got kinky twists put in. I wore these for about a month before I had a reality check. This was me and I needed to face the music. So, I took out the kinky twists and went to work for a week with my short curly afro. That's about all it took for me to get used to seeing myself with natural hair. Doing that made me realize that no one else truly cared about how I wear my hair. It was only my perception I had to contend with. After it grew to about three inches I started wearing it in two-strand twists and it started growing and growing. Soon I had long two-strand twists and my hair was thick and beautiful!

Best of all, it felt good. Wearing my hair in its natural state just felt good and still does. Up till this moment, I have never underestimated the importance and power of feeling good in life. In all aspects of life, feeling good is a high sign that you are in the right place. After three years of being natural, I permed it again. "Eyes rolling." That lasted for about two years and I cut it all off again and I've never looked back. That was at least ten years ago.

I like my natural hair. I love it. But it is a lot of work. The good things in life seem to be.

I wrote this book because too many black women know nothing about how to take care of their hair. We have been so indoctrinated into the straight hair aesthetic whether by perming, wigs, or weaves that we don't even know HOW to take care of our own hair. I don't want anyone with curly coarse hair to feel lost anymore. We do not have straight hair growing out of our heads and we cannot take care of it like it is straight.

As an expert in taking care of my curly hair, my goal now is to pass along my knowledge to my peers and the generations to come. I am excited to share my hair care routine and my styling routine with you. Learning how to take care of your hair is a form of self-love.

5
Basic Hair Care Routine

*T*his is a step-by-step guide to caring for your hair. I have low porosity and type four hair. I think that most African-Americans have this type of hair. I avoid products with silicones and use a clarifying shampoo with each wash. What I have learned is that hair care is scalp care. Keeping the scalp clean is paramount and therefore shampooing your hair every seven to ten days is the most important step to beautiful hair.

1. <u>Detangle hair with Oil and Water (warm)</u>. Section hair into large twists and **comb** through each section of hair from ends to roots. Wash day is the only day I use a comb on my hair.
2. <u>Rinse hair thoroughly with warm water</u>.
3. <u>Wash hair with shampoo</u>. Concentrate on the scalp. Use a shampoo that removes ALL build-up and dirt.
   (I DO NOT use sulfate-free shampoos because I need to eliminate all buildup from my scalp.)
4. <u>Rinse hair thoroughly with warm water</u>. Rinse all shampoo out of the hair
   (I sometimes do an ACV rinse with ¼ cup ACV and 1-quart water to ensure my scalp is squeaky clean) ACV-Apple Cider Vinegar
5. <u>Condition hair with a good deep conditioner</u>. Let it sit for about thirty minutes with a heated cap.
   (I use conditioners without silicones so that it can penetrate and soften my hair better. Silicones give the hair a

false sense of shine and silkiness that simply lays on top of the strands.)

6. <u>Rinse hair thoroughly with warm water</u>. Rinse all conditioner out of hair.
7. <u>Style hair with leave-in conditioner and oil</u>. Style in braids or twists. Let it air dry.
8. <u>Twenty-four (24) to forty-eight (48) hours later style hair again</u> using water, leave-in conditioner, oil, gels, grease, or whatever styling product you want for a long-lasting style.
9. <u>Wear this style for one or two weeks</u>, then repeat this routine.
10. <u>Spray your hair with water and seal it with oil</u> every other day until wash day.
11. <u>After you style</u>, you can wear a wig over your hair in braids, twists, or cornrows. Then, wear your hair loose a few days before your wash day.
12. <u>Oil your scalp</u> in between the parts and massage your scalp once or twice a week.

My Go-To Products

Go get these products today! They are very affordable.

My Basic Three

1. **Shampoo**- Head & Shoulders dry scalp 2 n 1
2. **Leave-in conditioner**- Cantu leave-in conditioning repair cream
3. **Oil**- olive oil- extra virgin

These three products alone will keep healthy hair on your head. Period. However, the basic three turns into The Basic Four when you realize that a good deep conditioner is worth the investment. Either of the two below will do. Find your Basic Three, moisturizing shampoo, leave-in conditioner, and oil, and keep them stocked. Do not compromise on your personal hair care.

The hair products below are some of my *Favorites* because I'm worth it!

Shampoo- Head & Shoulders dry scalp care 2 n 1, any Cantu shampoo that is not sulfate-free, Sulfur 8 shampoo

Oils- Extra virgin olive oil, grapeseed oil, castor oil, avocado oil

Grease- Blue magic hair grease, sulfur 8 medicated, Doo Gro medicated Anti-dandruff formula

Leave-in conditioner- Cantu leave-in conditioning repair cream, Camille Rose curl love moisture milk

Deep Conditioners: Camille Rose Algae Renew Deep Conditioner, Mielle Organics Babassu Oil & Mint Deep Conditioner.

Daily Spritz: Oyin handmade herbal hydration Greg Juice citrus lavender (green label)

If these products don't work, tons of other hair products will most likely work for your particular curl and texture. You will have to test and try them out to find the ones that work perfectly for you. I highly recommend every product that I listed for all hair types but if you don't like it, please find another one. I try different products from time to time but I always come back around to the basics listed above.

My Styling Method

You can style your hair in between washes. There are dozens of ways to style your hair. It simply depends upon your personal preferences. I recommend styling only once or twice in two weeks. This keeps your hands out of your hair which could cause breakage from too much manipulation. However, you can style it every day If you like.

For every style, this is the method to keep your hair moisturized.

First, fill a spray bottle with warm water

Secondly, Take down your hair one section at a time and spray with warm water

Third, put a generous amount of Cantu leave-in conditioner on that section of hair. Add leave-in to the entire length of hair with a heavy focus on the ends.

Fourth, let water and leave-in conditioner sit on the hair for about twenty seconds to allow it to soak in well.

Fifth, add your choice of oil or grease to the length of the hair to seal in the moisture. Heavy concentration on the ends of hair.

Sixth, detangle hair with your fingers, from ends to roots. Take your time and be gentle.

Seventh, now is the time to put whatever other styling products, gels, creams, lotions, etc., that you want on your hair.

Eighth, Re-braid or twists your hair or whatever style you are doing. Repeat this process for every section of hair.

Every day or couple of days spritz your hair with warm water and seal with an oil or grease.

The Way

I do things a certain way. This is probably the most important part of the book. Contrary to popular opinion, HOW you do things does matter. Below, I will share my tips and tricks as to why my hair routine works. This certain way adds to my hair's success and happiness.

- I section and detangle my hair before I wash it. I put it in large two-strand twists. This ensures that my hair will not tangle back up during the washing process. I use my olive oil mix (olive oil, avocado oil, and grapeseed oil) and water to detangle. Simple. Water= Slip, so I spray more water if I need the comb to slip through the section more easily.

- I wash my hair in the large twists sections that I put my hair into.

- I add a deep conditioner to each twisted section of hair and twist it back up. Again, Water = Slip. If my good deep conditioner isn't allowing my hair to slip through my fingers easily, I spray a bit of warm water on that section, and amazing, supreme slippage.

- I sit under a hooded dryer to deep condition every wash day for at least thirty minutes. The conditioner penetrates my hair texture better with heat, leaving it softer. Game changer.

- I wear my hair in braids(plaits) or twists for the entire two weeks in between my wash days. I'm confident in my appearance and I don't work a lot so I don't have to conform to society much. But remember you can always throw on a wig if you need to.

- I get my hair professionally straightened and my ends clipped every three months to ensure I have no split ends or single-strand knots in my hair.

- I always say "I love my hair."

6
The Bonus Tip

*Y*aass Hunny! There is a bonus tip. After ten years of working with my natural hair, my hair was healthy and long but it still stopped at a certain length. I would hear natural girls talk about their hair staying moist for three or four days after wash day, my hair was very dry after two days. My hair still shed more than I thought it should. I had a lot of single-stand knots at the ends of my hair and it was still frizzy even after I added all the products. When I would take my twists or plaits down to wear my hair out, it would take two or three days for it to fully plump out and be full and pretty.

One thing changed ALL of this. One product. One discovery. My holy grail product. I have always believed that there is one thing that can break the growth plateau or health plateau for every hair and I always hoped to find mine. Everyone has their own "peanut-butter solution" as I like to call it. (In reference to the 1985 film "The Peanut Butter Solution"). I would also like to credit the Youtuber 'Curly Proverbz' because she has been so informative and adventurous with herbs over the years. She is so positive about being able to grow your hair longer. I believe she has her own haircare line out now. As I said before, I do think my hair is very similar to the average African -American. So, my holy grail might just be yours too. So what is it? It's so simple. It's too easy. Most of you already have it in your cabinets right now. Many of us drink it every day. It's an herb. One of the healthiest herbs. Drumroll….. It's TEA. Active ingredient caffeine. Yes, Tea. Regular ole black tea. I use Earl Grey but I'm sure any variety will do. It stopped the shedding instantly literally. It stopped single-strand knots. My hair absorbs all of the products I put on it and stays moist for days. My cuticle lays much flatter, with no frizz! And my hair has shine and body! My hair is visibly longer and as soon as I take my twists or plaits down, my hair is plump and delicious and I can wear it out with confidence. It's crazy! Just from adding a tea rinse to my routine at the very end. Try it! You won't be disappointed.

How to use a Tea Rinse:
After all of the deep conditioner is rinsed out thoroughly, then do a final tea rinse.

Ingredients:
- Large bowl or bottle
- 1 pouch of earl grey tea
- 1 quart of distilled water

Place the tea bag in warm distilled water and let sit for about 30 minutes. Pour mixture over your hair and scalp and let sit for 15 seconds. Do not rinse out. Pat your hair dry with a cotton shirt or towel and style as usual.

For those who DO want to rinse the tea off, let it sit on your hair for about ten minutes, then rinse it off. I DO NOT advise anyone to leave the tea rinse in your hair UNTIL you know what your hair can and cannot tolerate. Tea is a **very strong herb** and one bag can irritate some scalps. Some might consider using more than one quart of water for better dilution. I have also used green tea and hibiscus tea successfully but I get the best results with black tea.

Tea can also irritate and scar your skin so be sure to wear a shirt that will cover your shoulders and chest and put a towel around your shoulders for the drippings.

That's it! Your hair will be stronger and stop shedding in a matter of minutes.

7
Conclusion

*I*n conclusion, having healthy hair is not about looking like everyone else. Even your hair in its healthiest state will not be appealing to someone. The goal is for YOU to like what you see. You know what healthy African American hair looks like and most importantly, what it feels like. Maintaining, handling, and styling African American hair textures is not easy but it is our duty. Most people have two or three features about their bodies that they don't like. This is not an excuse to hide it or cover it up. We must look at all of our features as a gift including our hair. God created us all and everything about us is purposeful. God gave us our hair for a reason and it is beautiful. Love your hair and love yourself. Wear your natural hair out for the world to see its glory. You are perfect just the way you are and so is your hair. Thank you for reading. I hope my words help and bless you.

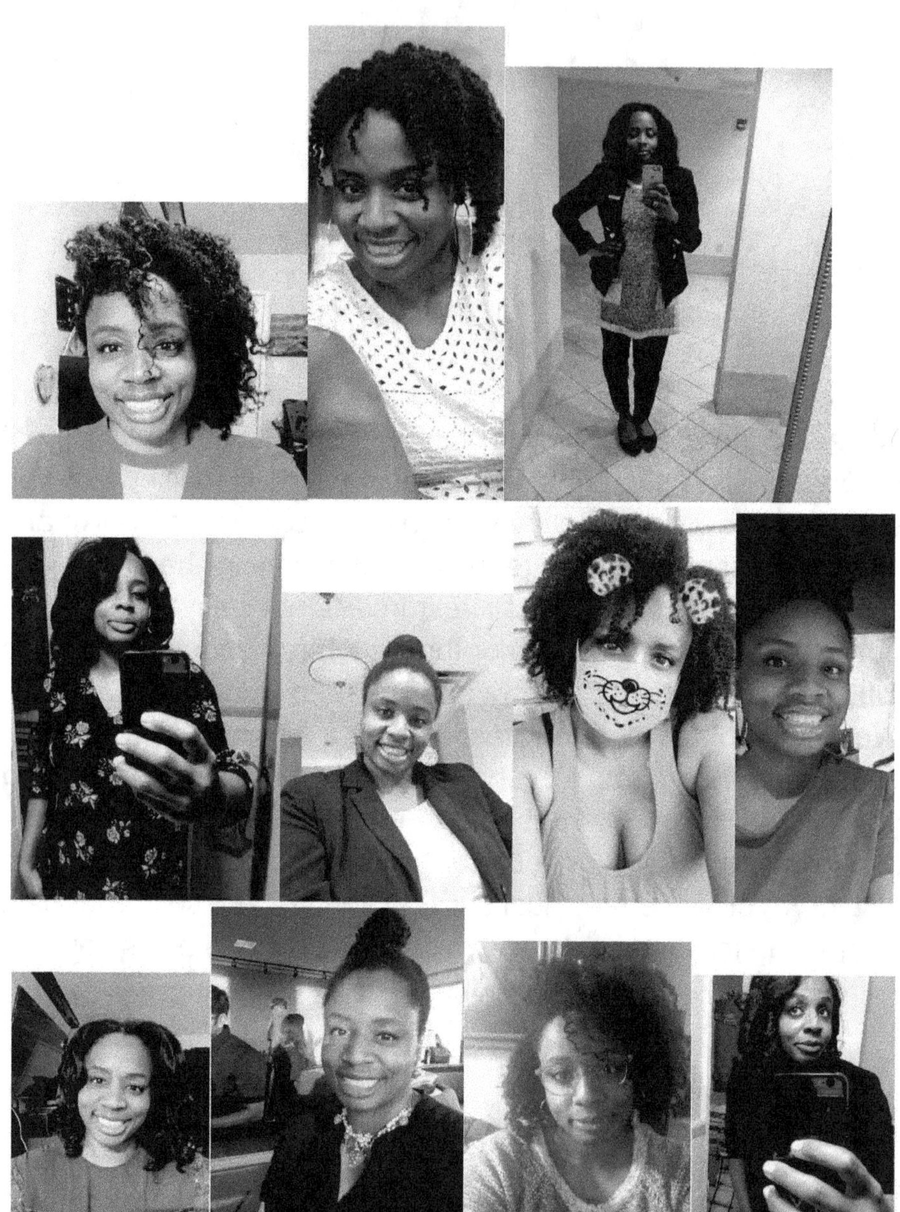

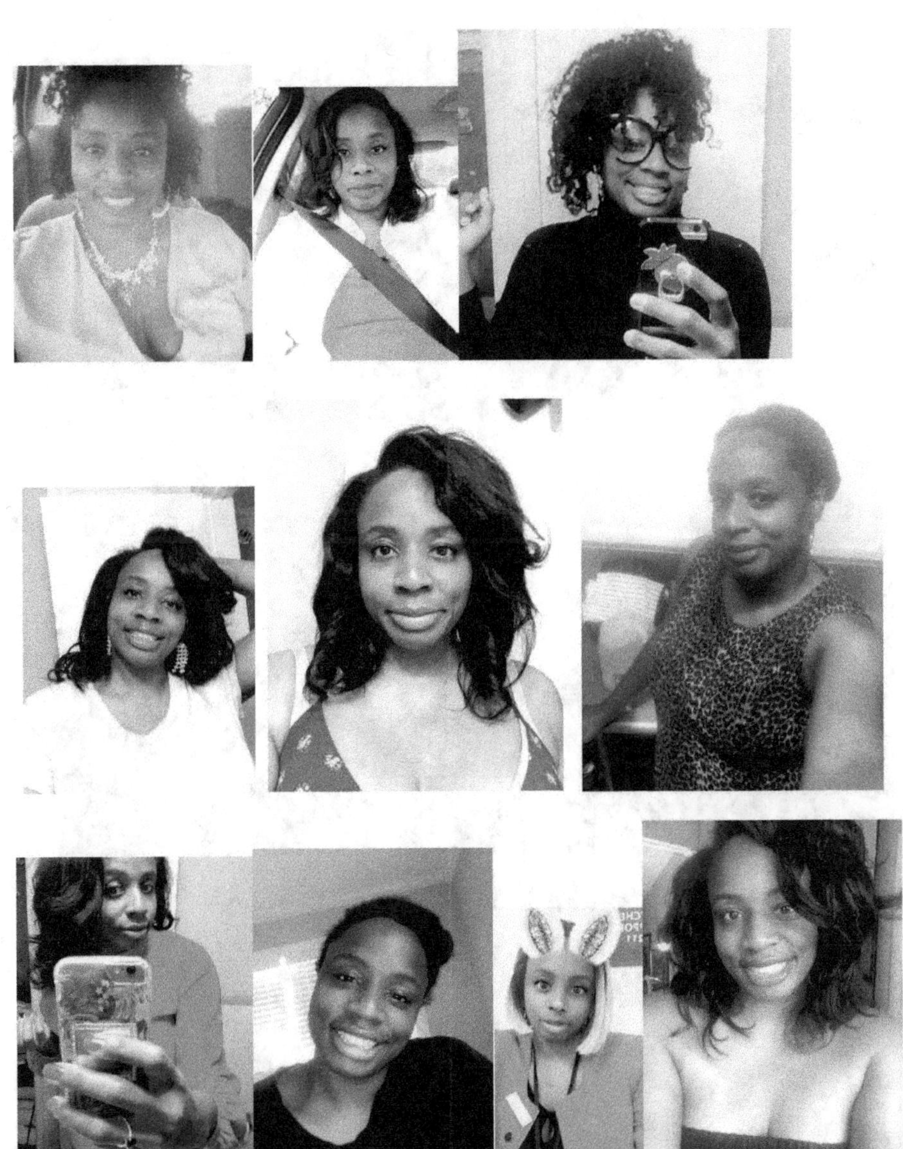

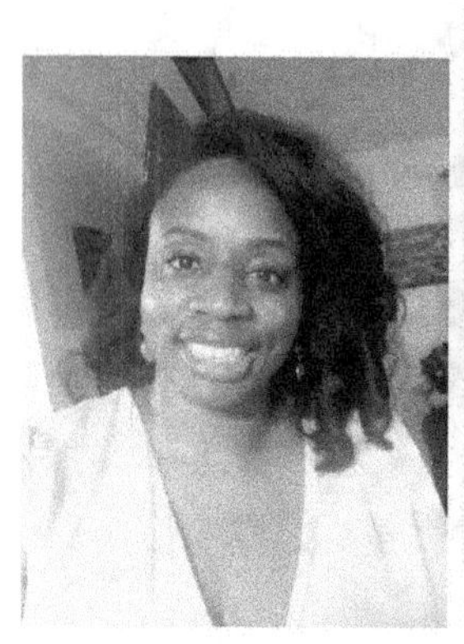
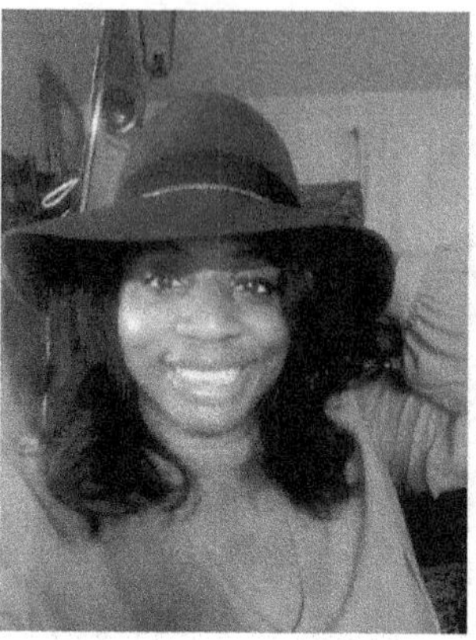
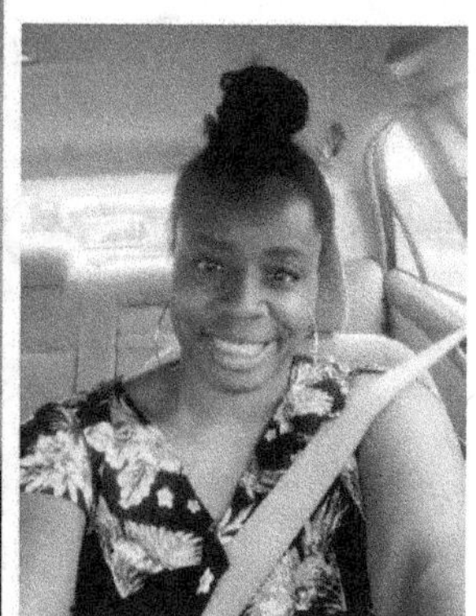
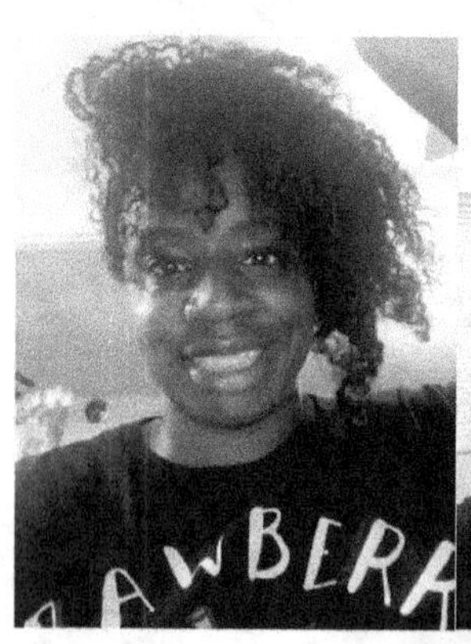
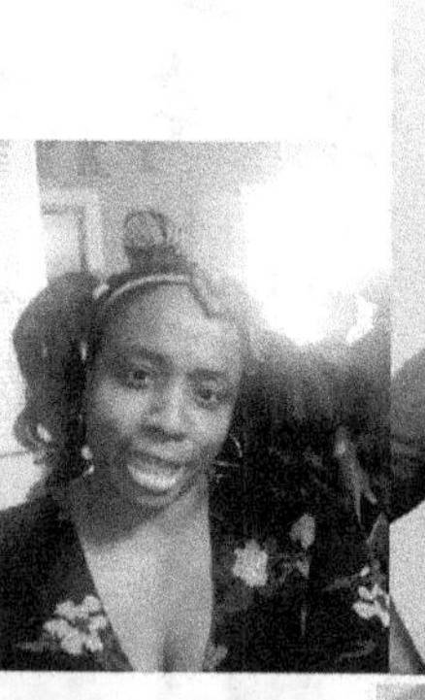
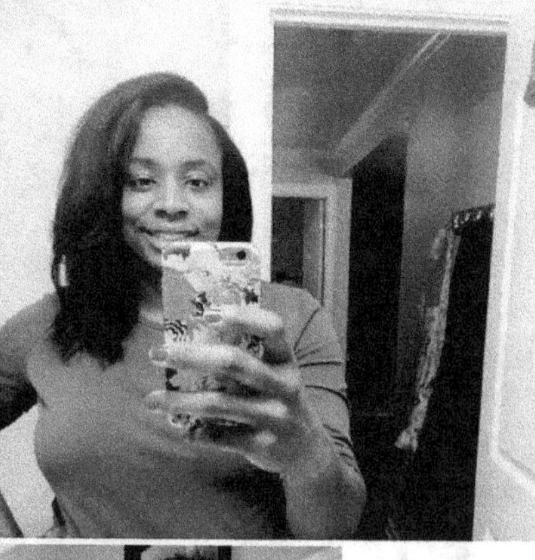
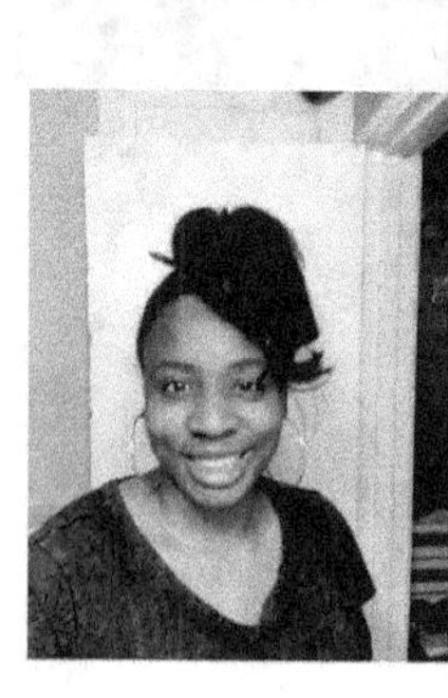
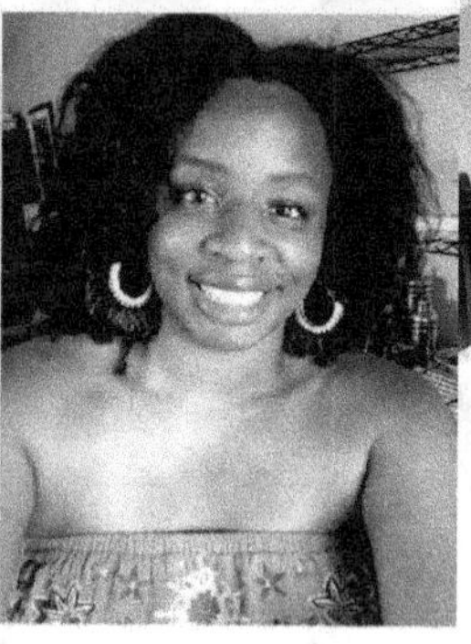
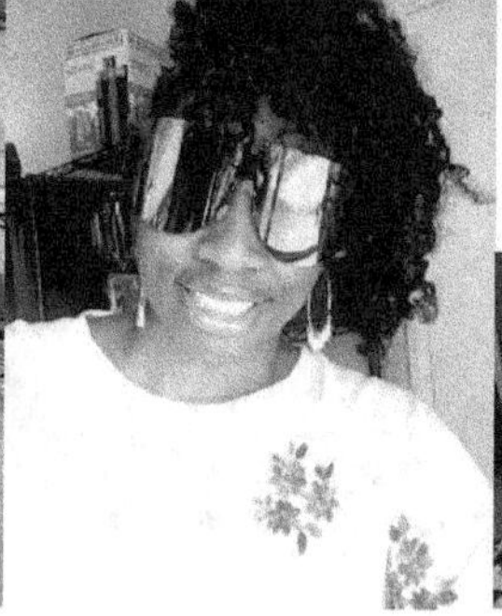
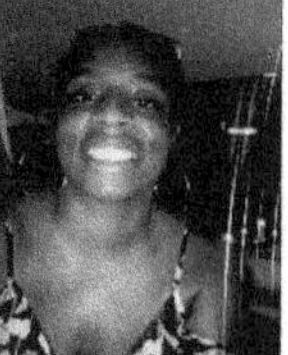